JUVENILE ARTHRITIS
The Mom's Story

Diane Kirkpatrick

Waterglen Press

Cover Art by Sue Kirkpatrick

Diane Kirkpatrick/Waterglen Press

Publisher's Note: This are the facts as I remember them. Names, characters, places, and incidents may have been changed slightly to protect the innocent. Locales and public names are sometimes used for atmospheric purposes. Book Layout © 2014 BookDesignTemplates.com

Juvenile Arthritis the Mom's Story/ Diane Kirkpatrick. -- 1st ed.

ISBN 978-1535144629

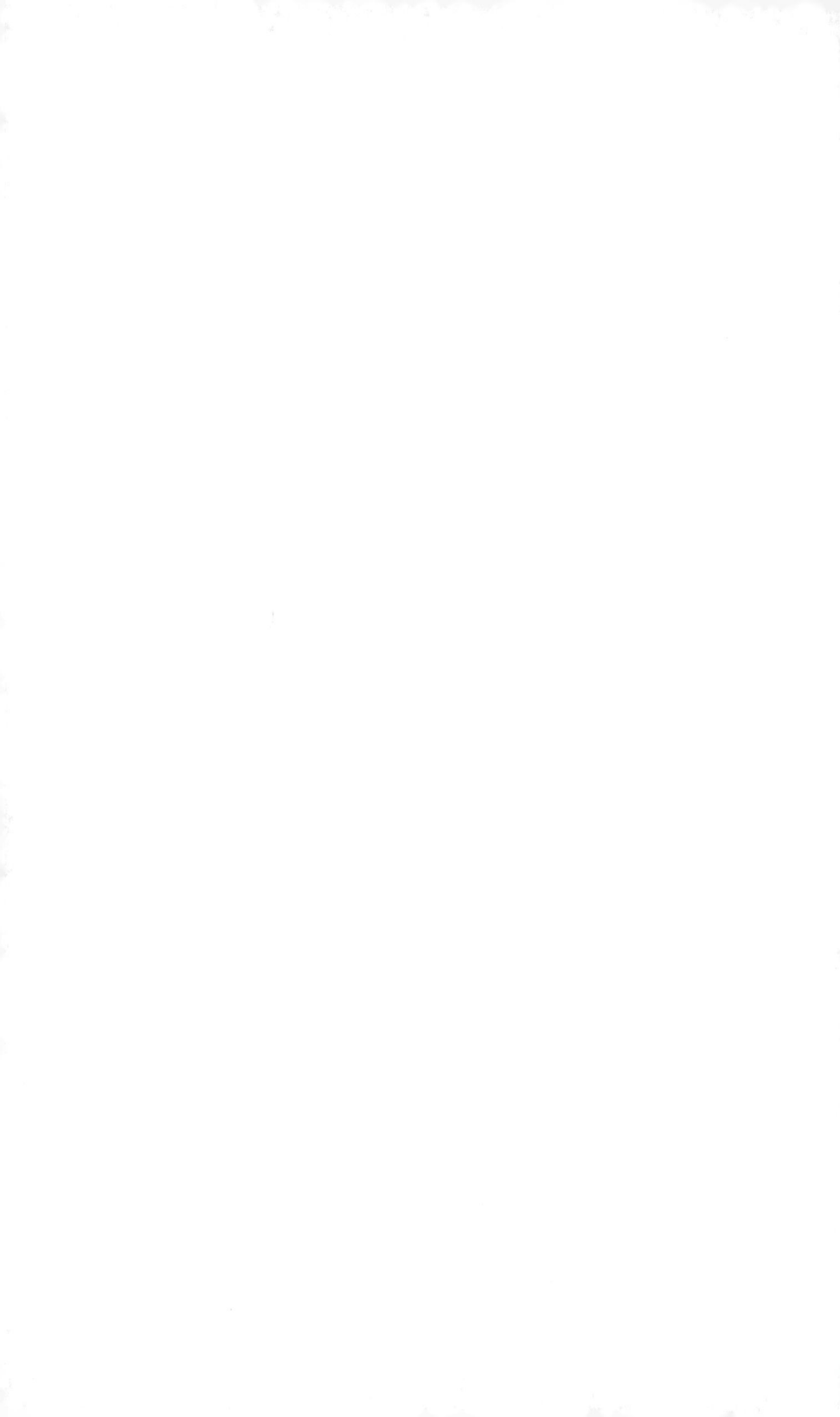

Contents

1 INTO

If you want to read cold, clinical, politically-correct descriptions, you can go to webmd.com.

After many revisions to this manuscript I decided that the only thing that makes this story interesting are my recollections of life as the mother of a chronically ill child. My son, Dan, had the pain of stiff and swollen joints. I had the pain of seeing him suffer and feeling like somehow it was my fault. So this story is more about me than my son.

At 7-years-old, my son was diagnosed with arthritis. I didn't even know that was possible.

I had so many questions and I felt so alone. Doctors seemed aloof. Friends and family didn't understand. Even the internet came up short. All the websites I found were clinical lists or drug company ads. I couldn't find any real, unedited experiences of juvenile arthritis.

After nearly a decade of dealing with this disease, I decided to write Dan's story. I wanted to make it as accurate as possible, so I searched through old clinic reports, lab results and the family calendar. As I dug up these facts, I also dug up a lot of memories. Some days I couldn't write because I was crying too hard with the painful recollections. Dan doesn't even remember most of it, which is ironic since most the anguish I felt was caused by my worry over Dan being robbed of normal childhood activities.

I don't mention my husband much in this book. It just becomes awkward to say my husband and I every other sentence. So I edited him out; sorry, Sam. I wanted to let you know that in most of these scenes my husband was either there or at home with the other kids. He was totally supportive and helpful. After a while we had a division of labor set up. I took kids to specialists and he took kids to the pediatrician for stitches, sore throats and check-ups. We did this so often that Dr. M (our regular pediatrician) didn't even know who I was. I once ended up at his office due to scheduling conflicts and Dr. M said he hadn't seen me at a his office in a long time. I groaned inwardly because I had been at the rheumatologist and ophthalmologist that week. Probably spending 10 hours driving to and seeing doctors.

Here is the thing about this book. I've re-written it nearly four times and I just want to be done. Kind of like I want to be done with this stupid disease. But I have a feeling that both of them are never going to fully go away.

2 PEDIATRICIAN

When Dan came down with the first symptoms of arthritis, I was severely distracted. I had just moved to a new house. I had five young children including a baby. I took care of this busy house while I worked part-time from home doing web programming.

One day, I was working on my computer when Dan got my attention. He was limping. And this concerned me because my active son is usually a ball of wild energy.

"Look at my fat toes," he said pointing to his bare foot.

I bent down to his foot so I could see better. His middle toes looked thicker than the others.

"Did you stub your toe?" I asked him.

"No it is just hurting," he said as he said as he sat on the floor so he hold his foot up closer to my face.

This was not the first time a child had come to me with a mysterious pain. I had a system for dealing with minor injuries like this.

"Put an ice pack on it."

"OK," he said and limped off to the freezer.

Everything was solved and I went about my business. It may have only been a few days later when Dan showed me a swollen ankle.

"I have already put an ice pack on it," he said as I examined it.

Again, I used my mom-skills and told him to wrap it in an ace bandage. I also gave him some children's Tylenol.

A few days later, both his ankles were swollen. Then his knees and fingers were red, swollen and hot to the touch. He walked around like an old man. I was running out of ace bandages and excuses.

When Dan said, "Hey look! I've got a cane like grandpa," I knew it was time to take him to the doctor.

Dan's pediatrician looked over my son's swollen fingers and toes. He watched Dan walk down the clinic hallway as he rubbed his chin in thought.

He asked me how long this had been going on.

"Maybe a couple months," I said, embarrassed. The way the doctor was acting made me think I should have brought him to the clinic before this.

"I think Dan has arthritis."

"But he is just a kid," I said.

"Kids can get arthritis," he explained. "His immune system is attacking his joints. I will get you an appointment with a pediatric rheumatologist."

Those two words didn't make sense together in my mind. But I was hopeful that if there was a specialist, then there was a treatment. I could get Dan help for this mysterious pain and swelling.

3 RHEUMATOLOGIST

Dan's swollen joints were worsening by the day. I was glad when we could finally get into see Dr. P, a pediatric rheumatologist at the children's hospital.

I had been to the children's hospital before with Dan's sister who had needed surgery for a birth defect. The maze of hallways with children's art and bubbling fish tanks brought back anxious memories.

By the time we were called back to the exam room, I had a hard time concentrating.

Dr. P asked questions in a thick accent as he examined Dan's joints.

"Have you given him any pain medication?" Dr. P asked.

"Not really," I said.

I had given Dan some children's Tylenol, but it never seemed to help. Then when I knew we were coming to see the doctor, I didn't want any medicine masking the symptoms. If I've learned anything about taking kids to the doctor, it is that only full symptoms get full treatment.

"Made him tough it out eh?"

I felt defensive about that so I just nodded.

"Can you make a claw?" Dr. P asked as he showed Dan how to curve his fingers.

Dan tried to imitate Dr. P's bent hand, but Dan's swollen fingers couldn't do it. I also made a claw-hand behind my back just to make sure I was OK too.

"These swollen fingers are sometimes called sausage fingers and they are common in juvenile arthritis," the doctor said.

I would have replied but I didn't want to distract Dr. P while he made marks on a skeleton diagram in his notes. He had marked the toes, ankles, knees, wrists, and fingers.

"Since he has more than 15 affected joints, he has polyarticular arthritis," the doctor offered.

That wasn't the diagnosis I had expected. I had been looking up rheumatoid arthritis on the internet. I didn't want to sound like I thought I knew more than a doctor.

"Does that mean he has rheumatoid arthritis?" I clarified.

"We won't know until we do blood tests."

"What kind of tests?"

"The tests will tell us if he is having an immune response, if he has RA factor, and if his liver is functioning normally."

"Do you need those results before you can treat him?" I asked.

"You can give him an anti-inflammatory medication. I will write a prescription for liquid naproxen. It takes a few months for the medication to take full effect. If he isn't improving in a few weeks, let me know." Dr. P said.

I didn't like hearing how long he would have to wait for relief. I also felt frustrated that I would have to call for more answers. I wish I could get the good remedies while we are here at the hospital.

"Is he going to get better?" I asked.

"Don't worry about that. We will find something to help him."

I left the clinic with a stack of papers, prescriptions and lab test orders. The papers described arthritis symptoms and clinic policies. The policies scared me a little because they required you to be so prepared and I felt like my brain was scattered all over the place after listening to the doctor.

4 LABORATORY TESTS

In my former life, before kids, I had been a lab tech. I remember learning to draw blood from babies and kids. The tiny babies would scream and scream as you milked precious blood out of their tiny heels. I hated it. I could only dread having to watch my son go through that. I comforted myself with the thought that Dan was not a baby. He was tough. Maybe tougher than I was.

The clinic seemed to be miles from the hospital laboratory. Dan and I walked through corridors. I hated the child-made art that decorated the walls. Stressed parents pulling sick children in red, plastic wagons clogged the hallways. Was I now one of them again?

I found the waiting room for the lab. It was full of tired and cranky toddlers and babies. Dan thought it would be fun to try to play one of the PlayStation games. Our LEGO people ran in circles until I convinced Dan the controls were broken.

"When can we go home?" he asked.

"Soon. We have to do some tests," I said. My mind flew to thoughts of his baby sisters, traffic, insurance, prescriptions and the fact that I was starving.

"What do you think of this toy?" I picked up one of the toys from a basket full of them. I didn't even care if there were hospital germs on it.

He looked at it for a minute and then continued to complain. I wanted to scold him and tell him to stop whining. But then I felt sorry for him because he had arthritis.

I distracted him with a different toy. I thought about preparing him for the idea of blood tests, but then I looked at the other parents and kids within earshot and decided that this might not be the best time or place. I'm sure the techs will help him understand. They work at a children's hospital after all.

The lab tech called Dan's name and we went back behind the counter to a draw room. They helped him sit in a chair and then folded a small table down in front. I don't remember what we talked about, but the phlebotomist was good and Dan hardly flinched as he drew 5 or 6 tubes of blood from his small hand.

"Way to go buddy!" the tech said as he gave Dan a high five. "Now let's find the prize drawer."

Dan followed the tech to the drawer where Dan took 5 minutes choosing the best dollar-store prize. He had already forgotten about the needle.

5 WAITING FOR ANSWERS

Dan did not improve. Even though I had taken Dan to the specialist, gotten prescriptions and lab tests, his symptoms were the same or worse. But at least I knew what we were dealing with. His mysterious pain was not going to kill him in the next month. Some of my fears were quieted but some were made worse. I still wasn't sure what I could do besides force him to take liquid naproxen every day.

I tried to make him more comfortable. I helped him get around and I let him ride in the special shopping carts at the store. I bought him more ace bandages because he thought those were cool.

I would not normally have taken anyone on a long car trip in his condition, but unfortunately we had to drive to Canada the next month for my husband's grandfather's funeral. The trip was 700 miles. We stopped often in order to try to make it easier on Dan.

We hardly ever see the Canadian relatives and they were all very concerned about Dan's swollen joints. I felt like I had to explain about his problem over and over again.

Maybe it was good that we didn't change our vacation plans to accommodate Dan. We still went to reunions and the lake and the swimming pool even if I had to carry Dan in order to do it. I hope it made life more normal for everyone, but sometimes I think it just made everyone cranky.

6 BACK TO THE RHEUMATOLOGIST

I returned to the rheumatologist with Dan a month later. I was excited to finally get more answers. I wanted to get different medicine because the naproxen didn't seem to be helping.

Dr. P carefully examined each of Dan's swollen joints as he compared his notes.

"He has more joints involved now," he said.

"I know. And the joints seem more swollen than before," I offered. I didn't want him to think that Dan was improving. Because he wasn't and if you are getting worse maybe you can get better drugs and with better drugs, maybe Dan could start to lead a normal life.

"The RA factor was inconclusive, but his white blood cell count was high."

I was a laboratory technologist 15 years ago and I know that white blood cells are elevated for an infection or other inflammatory process like arthritis. But if you look at Dan's joints you can tell there is inflammation without a blood test. I decided that I won't reveal my background to the doctor because maybe I can get more information that way. Plus, I could be wrong.

"What does that mean?"

"His immune system is attacking his joints, but we don't know why."

"So it is rheumatoid arthritis?"

"It is idiopathic. That means we don't know what is causing it. Sometimes you just don't know what is causing the joints to swell."

I sighed. That did not sound good.

The doctor kept reviewing the notes and then offered, "One interesting result is that he is HLA B27 positive. HLA B27 is an antigen on the red blood cell that suggests a greater risk of developing an autoimmune disease. Not everyone with HLA B27 gets arthritis, but it helps confirm a diagnosis. If you have that marker, the disease progresses more slowly, but it also doesn't respond to treatment as quickly."

"Does that mean we have to wait longer for different treatment?"

"No, since he didn't respond to anti-inflammatory medicine, we can start him on methotrexate. With his diagnosis we have to start one medicine at a time and give each one a chance to work. I will ramp things up slowly. If he had rheumatoid arthritis I could give everything at once."

"Does methotrexate come in a liquid?" I ask, thinking about how Dan is too young to swallow pills.

"It is an injection. We will teach you to give it to him at home." Then he looks at Dan and says, "I bet you can even do it yourself."

"Yeah," Dan said even though I didn't think he had been paying attention to what the doctor had been saying. I didn't even know what to think about an injectable medication. I was speechless.

"Methotrexate has certain side-effects that are less if you take it as an injectable. This medicine has been around for a long time so it shouldn't be too expensive. You know it used to be used to treat cancer. But for arthritis treatment you use much lower doses. I think we will start with a .5 ml dose."

The doctor went to get the medical assistant that came in the exam room to teach Dan how to give the injection. It seemed like a quick instruction. I'm glad they also gave me some hand-outs so I could remember some of the steps at home.

7 FIRST INJECTION

The medicine came in a glass vial with a pack of 10 small needles. I carefully read the instruction the doctor had given me and collected other supplies I might need. I got alcohol prep pads, a sharps container and tiny circle bandages.

My house is usually full of childish energy as Dan and his sisters laugh as they play or cry when they fight. I knew I needed quiet if this injection was going to go well. I put all of Dan's sisters to bed, or at least in their rooms before starting.

I spread the supplies on the kitchen table and reviewed all the instructions with Dan carefully. I wanted to get this right since I had never given a shot before.

I wiped the top of the methotrexate vial with an alcohol pad. Then I filled the tiny syringe.

"Stop," Dan said, "I want to do it myself."

Dr. P had said Dan could do the injection if he was supervised. I thought I could do this better and faster but I hesitated. I knew it would be good for Dan to take some control of his disease so I gave him the pre-filled syringe.

Dan sat on a kitchen chair turned sideways, his elbow resting on the table. He held the syringe over his leg.

I reminded him to pinch his thigh and then stick the needle in quickly. Next I rubbed alcohol on his leg to prepare the skin. He coughed and gagged a little.

"What's wrong?"

"I hate that smell. Why did you do that?"

"I need to make sure you don't get an infection from the shot. The alcohol cleans the germs off the skin."

Dan sighed and tried to be strong. I sat in another kitchen chair to supervise.

Dan held the syringe over his thigh for 5 minutes.

"Just do it," I encouraged.

"Not yet," he said

My patience was wearing thin as he waited another 5 minutes.

"Do you want me to do it?"

"No"

Finally, after 20 minutes of encouraging and nagging him, he finally stuck the needle in his leg. He pushed the plunger almost imperceptibly slow.

When he was done he gave me the syringe which I disposed of. Then I put a tiny band aid on the small mark made by the needle.

Then Dan threw-up in the kitchen trash can.

Alarmed that Dan might be having a reaction to something, I read over the notes from the doctor.

"Are you OK?"

"I'm just nauseous."

I have him sip a little peppermint water and then send him off to bed to maybe sleep off the nauseous feeling.

8 PHYSICAL THERAPY

The methotrexate injections were going well except for the occasional nausea. But now that we knew what to expect I was prepared with peppermint and a trash can in case he was very nauseous. But even with the new medicine, Dan was not improving much.

A neighbor suggested that I take Dan to physical therapy. She could only sing the praises of how physical therapy had helped her shoulder feel better.

I asked the rheumatologist about it and he was not enthusiastic.

"Maybe he can build up his muscles so his joints won't hurt so much," I offered.

Dr. P looked through his notes. "It shouldn't hurt anything," he said. "His pain is caused by an immune response, but I guess you never know."

"Do you recommend anyone?"

Dr. P gave me a paper with some addresses. One address was in a nearby town so I made an appointment for Dan. When I saw the office, it seemed geared to children much younger than Dan, but I was hopeful anyway.

"What are your therapy goals?" the therapist asked my son.

Dan didn't answer. I wondered if he was paying attention. After a few moments of silence, I took over. "He wants to walk half a block without pain," I said.

Dan nodded and then added, "I want to be able to ride my scooter."

My eyes watered. It was not fair that my little son was worried about that kind of thing. I hid my teary eyes by pretending to blow my nose.

"Let me watch you walk up and down the hall," the therapist said.

Dan limped down the hall while the therapist made notes. After that, Dan rode a stationary bike and then practiced some stretches.

I asked the therapist if he had any suggestions for Dan's pain.

"Try warm, moist heat. Foot baths may help his ankles."

"What about his wrists and hands?"

The therapist thought for a minute.

"Have you ever see one of those hand spas with wax in it? Dip his hand in the wax and then put an oven mitt over it. The warmth will make his wrists feel better."

I nodded my head because I liked those ideas. I found an antique footbath at the thrift store. It could hold so much water it would cover his ankles. I also bought a hand bath. Dan and his sisters had too much fun with the hand wax. Wax ended up all over the kitchen table and walls.

I was diligent with Dan's physical therapy program but I could never get Dan to admit that any of my efforts were helping. His pain continued to get worse. When I got the $300 bill for the physical therapy appointment, I decided we would have to stick with home therapy.

9 INCREASED METHOTREXATE

Dan continued the methotrexate injections every week. Now that we knew what to expect, they weren't as bad. The alcohol smell still made him gag.

"I hate that smell!" he said every time.

My strategy was to fill the syringe in the other room. When I had to wipe his skin with the alcohol, he held his nose while it dried Then I would throw it away in a trash can in a different room.

"I'm going to invent an alcohol prep pad that doesn't smell," he told me once. He was always thinking about inventions at this age.

At the next appointment I told Dr. P, "He is taking all the medicine, but he isn't getting any better."

Dr. P examined Dan's joints again. "Less joints are involved," he said because his fingers and toes were less swollen than before.

"But his ankles and knees are worse, and he is in a lot of pain when he walks," I countered.

"We could increase the methotrexate."

My heart sank, "more injections?"

"No, just increase the amount to .7 ml."

"Is there any other way to give methotrexate? The shots are awful. It takes hours to finish one."

"I'm sorry, the injections have fewer side effects. I will have a child life specialist come talk to you about making the injections go better."

Dr. P gave me the prescription and then told us to wait in the exam room. I wondered what a child life specialist was a politically-correct name for.

After a few minutes, a cute young girl came in the room. She was carrying a basket full of games. Dan looked over the games. Most of them looked too babyish for his taste.

The girl dug through the games and found a little, round gadget.

"This is a 20-questions game. Play this while you give yourself the injection."

We all tried out the game a few times and Dan thought it was fun.

"If you use this while giving the injection, it will be a distraction. Then it won't be so bad," she told Dan.

Dan played the game during the entire hour-long ride home from the clinic. He played it with his sisters. He played the game through the injections. But they still took hours, but now I had to play this dumb game at the same time.

10 SIDE EFFECTS

With the bigger dose of methotrexate, Dan's joint pain finally started to decrease. Over the next few weeks, he began to walk more. He went to karate class and joined a soccer team.

But then the side-effects showed up.

My little chatterbox was silent. I thought he was depressed. But then I realized he had developed huge mouth sores. They were so painful he couldn't talk.

What a terrible trade-off. Either he could walk or he could talk.

I called the clinic about the mouth sores.

"He has so many blisters inside his mouth, he won't talk," I told the nurse.

Later that day the nurse called me to tell me to increase the folic acid dose. "It is a common side effect of methotrexate," she said.

Dan had been taking folic acid since he had started the methotrexate as a way help his body deal with side effects. I thought they had been talking about nausea. So I gave him double the amount now, 2 pills.

This strategy did not make a difference with the mouth sores.

I asked our dentist if he had any suggestions. He gave us some "Magic Mouthwash" but that didn't help either.

My little boy was suffering again.

At the next rheumatologist appointment, I show Dr. P the mouth sores. He quizzed me about if Dan took the folic acid.

I assured him we were doing all we could.

"We should decrease the methotrexate back to .5 ml," he said.

So over the next month, with less methotrexate, his mouth sores healed, but his joint pain got worse.

11 ENBREL

Another month goes by and Dan's joints are still swollen. Dr. P was finally convinced the methotrexate and naproxen weren't strong enough.

"Is there anything else we can do?" I asked him.

"I think he should start Enbrel. Enbrel is a biologic response modifier. That means it fights the cause of the arthritis, not just the symptoms."

"That sounds promising," I said. But at the same time I wondered why we didn't just start with that medication.

"Yes, many of the new drugs are amazing."

Dr. P writes notes in Dan's chart which has become pretty thick after nearly of year of visits.

"Does it come as a liquid?"

"It is a weekly injection."

My heart sank. Dan hated getting injections and I hate giving them.

"It is a little more expensive, but I think Dan should try it," the doctor said.

I agreed. Wouldn't I pay anything to help Dan? This is what I was waiting for. I left the clinic with more hope than I had felt in a long time.

That evening, I called Walgreens to see if I could order Enbrel for Dan. I gave them my insurance information. After more than a few transfers, a pharmacist comes on the line.

"We can get Enbrel, but we can't bill medically," the man said. "Your insurance will only cover injectable medicine as a procedure. You should try a hospital pharmacy."

After more calls, I found a network hospital pharmacy that could bill our insurance correctly. I later went to pick up the medicine and was shocked when the bill was $400.

"How many doses are in here?" I asked as I held up the snazzy reusable insulated container that came with the medicine. I wasn't sure about medicine that came with swag.

"That should last a month," the pharmacist said.

I swallowed and put the total on the credit card. It would be worth it if it helped Dan walk again.

"Keep the Enbrel in the fridge until a few hours before injection. It is best to give the shot at room temperature," the tech instructed.

That evening, I prepared Dan and then carefully gave him the room-temperature, pre-filled, glass syringe. He held the needle over his leg for long moments before injecting it. Again, he pushed the plunger so slowly it was almost undetectable by the human eye.

"Why are you going so slowly?"

"It stings," he said.

"But if you go faster, it will be over sooner," I begged. I wanted this to be over because I was getting tired and wanted to go to bed.

"No," he said.

We had the same argument every time he gave himself an injection. He would not go faster and I didn't feel like

I could take that control away from him. He was the one suffering from the disease. I couldn't help him feel better so I could suffer through these medication sessions as some kind of penance. It was so tempting to reach over and push the plunger and get the whole thing over with.

After a half hour, Dan said, "I have a funny taste in my mouth."

I sat at the kitchen table with my head down, waiting. I kept the trash can close in case he was nauseous.

One hour later, he was finally finished. At least I didn't have to play the 20 questions game.

"We will have to do methotrexate tomorrow, I'm too tired tonight," I said.

12 SUPPORT SYSTEM

I'm not sure where to put this part of the story so we are going to take a little intermission while I rant about the kind of support I received during these first years. (Except for my amazing husband of course.)

And in order to really understand my point of view, you have to understand my past. I was raised in the Mormon church, a fundamentalist religion. I was a devout believer throughout my childhood and through this point of my life.

There were some benefits to this belief. I had a ready-made community that could support me. I could have had plenty of free casseroles. Mormons love to bring casseroles. Of course, casseroles don't help much since my kids were picky eaters. If I accepted dinners, I would still have to cook for my kids anyway and then return the neighbors' dishes too.

Another benefit is that the church has a food pantry that poor members can use if they get the permission of the bishop. We were able to use this for a while because we were so poor due to large medical bills.

One drawback was that church teaching about faith-healing. If you are good enough, then you can be healed from your sickness. So many people would talk about how they prayed and God healed them. So since my son was not getting better, I felt like I wasn't good enough.

A good Mormon shows their faith by working hard at perfectly obeying the rules. When things don't go perfectly in your life, you need to examine how you could be better.

I was scrupulous about keeping the many Mormon commandments. I tried so hard to be perfect, I was wearing myself out. I was getting up at 5:00 a.m. so I could get all the scripture reading, praying, temple service and cooking and cleaning that a perfect Mormon mom is expected to do. Plus I was staying up late to work or help with homework. Anytime I had a minute to just sit, I immediately fell asleep.

The church members, many of whom were my neighbors, did not understand why my son was not running and playing like a normal child. They let me know that I should make sure Dan didn't eat any sugar or gluten. They suggested essential oil rubbed on his skin or diffused in the air. It was like they just assumed I wasn't doing everything possible to figure out how to help my son.

The youth activities that my son should have participated in rarely took his condition into account so he couldn't do many activities with his friends. The bishop chided me for not letting Dan go on scout camp-outs. Even after describing his immunosuppressant state and the fact that sleeping on the cold ground would worsen his symptoms the next day, he just shook his head and told me I didn't have enough faith.

I'll never forget the time one neighbor called me on the phone to ask me what medication Dan was taking. No one ever called me on the phone to ask a question so specific so I was kind of in shock at her boldness.

"Is Dan on Enbrel?" she asked.

After I admitted he was on the drug, she began to rant about the pharmaceutical industry.

"That medicine is made by the greediest medical company. They make so much money from that medication, it is sinful."

"It is the only medicine that has made any difference," I said.

"It has so many side effects. You just need to makes sure he eats clean. Have you tried physical therapy or essential oils?"

I listened to her drone on and on. I wish I had just hung up on her. I just can't even imagine a person thinking they should call a young, harried mother of a chronically ill child and tell them they are doing something wrong. Am I really supposed to tell this child, who is suffering in pain that he can't eat any treats? Seriously?

What about extended family support? I wish I had been more vocal about what I needed help with. It was just so hard to explain what would be helpful because I didn't know. Rather than try to direct people, it was easier to keep everyone distant.

Maybe I didn't deal with the disease as well as I could. Maybe I was too sensitive. Maybe I should have communicated better. But I'm not going to go there. I try to look on my past self with compassion. When my son got arthritis, I had it too. I was in pain and didn't know it. And you know what? I did a hell of a job under the circumstances.

Do you know someone that struggles with a chronically ill child? Here are some ways to actually help.

1. Babysit her other children while she had to take the sick child to the doctor.

2. Give her money.

3. Tell her she is doing a good job.

4. Tell her she is a good mom.

DO NOT offer advice. Really, just don't do it. Even if you think it will help, don't offer advice. Even if the mom asks for advice, don't give any advice!

13 INACTIVE DISEASE

Dan's symptoms are finally fading. I didn't like adding another weekly injection, but the new medicine worked like a miracle. Somehow we were able to find ways to pay for the expensive drug. I usually put the bill on the credit card because I thought going into debt for the expensive drug was 100% worth it. Dan was acting and playing like any other child his age.

Three years after his first diagnosis, Dan was symptom free. The rheumatologist began to decrease Dan's medicine. First he decreased the dose of methotrexate and then when the symptoms stayed away, he stopped it entirely. Then he stopped the Enbrel and naproxen, until eventually Dan had no medication.

"You never get cured. We call his disease inactive," the doctor explained.

"Do you think it will come back?"

"It is hard to say. Maybe a 50-50 chance."

I was ready and willing to take that chance.

I loved watching Dan be active and pain-free. I enjoyed the extra room in the budget without the medical bills.

I dared to believe that arthritis was behind us.

14 INJURY

Dan was symptom-free for nearly a year. Maybe I was getting too confidant. But the pain-free interlude came to a sudden end.

We were on a family trip to the library when Dan was about 11-years-old. As we walked to the car through the library parking lot, Dan was running, arms swinging, teasing his sisters and not paying attention. I remember feeling glad he was so happy and carefree.

But then I heard a thud as he fell to the ground, crying.

"What happened?" I asked as I knelt over him, asking him what happened.

"I hit my knee," he said as he pointed to the fender of a parked car.

I comforted him while I snuck a look at the fender of the indicated car. The way he acted there should be a large dent there. I didn't see anything.

I helped Dan to our van since he couldn't put any weight on his injured leg.

I didn't really think much of the injury. It seems my kids are especially clumsy and I am always handing out ice packs and ace bandages. But after I give them sympathy and attention, they quickly forget about the temporary pain.

But over the next few hours, his knee swelled double in size.

It reminded me of his arthritic knees. But it couldn't be arthritis. Would that start with an injury? I figured it had to be some kind of bruise but he continued to limp and complain for weeks. Then his ankles began hurting. With a sick feeling in my stomach, I made an appointment with the rheumatologist.

15 STEROIDS

The rheumatologist was not happy to see Dan return to the clinic. I felt embarrassed as I explained to the doctor that Dan's joints were swollen and painful again.

"Any history of injuries or fevers?"

The doctor frowned as I told him about the story of the library parking lot. I explained how I had treated the injury and that I had given anti-inflammatories.

"Sometimes a round of prednisone can stop flare-ups like this," he said as he wrote a prescription.

The prednisone didn't help the pain, but Dan felt the side-effects. For the next few weeks, Dan had painful joints, swollen cheeks and red, blotchy skin. When Dan did not improve, I called the clinic and was given a prescription for even more prednisone.

Finally a month later, the rheumatologist recommended methotrexate.

I did not want to have to go through all the medicines again before finding some pain relief for Dan. I explained to the doctor that Enbrel was the only thing that helped last time.

"It is the protocol. We can start Enbrel next month."

I was mentally preparing for the extra cost of Enbrel in the shrinking family budget. I was willing to pay any cost to help Dan feel better, but there had to be another way. Maybe

I could get it from Mexico or Canada or something. I got so much spam about getting cheaper Viagra from a foreign country. Maybe those junk emails were based on a sliver of fact. It would probably be cheaper to go out of the country and get it.

Trying to feel out whether international travel would be an option I asked, "Is there any way to get cheaper Enbrel?"

"You didn't have the payment assistance program last time? That is a shame," the doctor says as he shakes his head.

"No," I said as my heart went cold. Why didn't anyone tell me? Why didn't the insurance company or clinic say anything? I blamed myself because I never asked the right question. What if I still wasn't asking the right questions? Would I ever figure this out? I felt horrible because payment assistance would have made our lives so much better a couple years ago.

Big lesson learned: expensive medicine usually has payment assistance but you have to ask for it. And no one is required to tell you.

16 INEFFECTIVE MEDICINE

I signed up for the payment assistance program for Enbrel the next month when the rheumatologist finally prescribed it again. I didn't feel so much pressure about the costs as I dutifully supervised Dan's injections.

I carefully warmed each vial of medicine only 2 hours before each injection. I had a big check list of all the medicine I had to give so I would not forget them. I had piroxicam, folic acid, methotrexate and Enbrel to keep track of.

I thought if I went the extra mile, I could get Dan feeling better. I felt more desperate because this flare-up was hitting even worse than his first attack of arthritis. His knees, ankles, hands and wrists were painful and swollen. He could not do school work. He rarely played or even walked. Many days he just wanted to stay in bed and moan.

My heart was breaking for him.

I don't understand the people who thought I was babying him. Would a child really fake pain enough that they stayed in bed? I've been around enough children to know that the natural state of childhood is energy and excitement. I was doing everything the doctor told me to do.

So I dedicated more free time and money to his care. He not only endured the injections and pills, he had to put up with my renewed zeal for physical therapy. He endured foot baths, essential oil massages, hand wax treatments and flexibility training. I tried it all, but Dan's pain and swelling worsened.

I blamed myself. I blamed God and sometimes I blamed Dan. I was not as patient as I could have been. I was barely keeping it together some days.

Dan could not walk anywhere and I was tired of his excuses. I borrowed an old, broken wheelchair from my parent's attic. It was too big and so heavy, but it was all I could afford.

"The medicine is not working," I told the doctor after a few months of waiting.

"Give it time," he said.

So we waited some more while my son was suffering. I was suffering.

17 UVEITIS

One day, Dan said, "My eyes hurt."

I examined his eyes. They looked red as if he had conjunctivitis.

"It is probably just pink-eye. I have some medicine for that," I said as I put some drops in his eyes from a previous pink-eye diagnosis. I didn't really think anything about it because as a mom, this happened all the time.

A few days later, Dan got my attention again. "My eyes still hurt."

I shined a light at this eyes to examine them more closely. They were just as red as when I had first looked at them. They should have been better by now.

"Ow," he said, "That's too bright,"

"You are stalling again. Go do your homework." It seemed like Dan had so many things wrong with him, I had to draw the line somewhere.

Dan had obediently gone to his desk to work but I noticed he was wearing sunglasses.

"Why are you wearing sunglasses to do your homework?"

"The light hurts my eyes," Dan said.

Then I remembered that JIA kids can get some complications in their eyes. We had been going to the ophthalmologist yearly because of the potential for complications. We had just been a couple months ago and he didn't have any problems. I looked in the fat folder full of hand-outs from the clinic. I finally found the information about eye problems. The chart indicated that kids with HLA-B27 didn't have much of a risk.

But then I noticed the asterisk. The footnote said that if they ever have red, painful eyes, to see a doctor as soon as possible.

Now I begin to panic. What if Dan is going blind?

I called the ophthalmology clinic and tried to get more information. I described Dan's painful, red eyes and asked if it was serious. The nurse seemed unconcerned and would not make an appointment for my son closer than 3 months out.

"Is there anyone that he can see sooner? I think it might be serious. He has juvenile arthritis."

"I'm sorry We'll call you back if something opens up."

When they didn't call after 2 days, I called them again.

"Is there anyone that can just take a look at his eyes? Maybe a local optometrist?"

I was thinking that guy at the local Walmart had to have one of those eye microscopes.

"I don't think that is a good idea."

"Then what should I do?"

"I don't know, ma'am."

I think I was so frustrated that I didn't handle this well. I cried at the receptionist, "This could be really serious!"

I try not to blame the receptionist when I think of this incident. She was probably only a teenager and following protocol. But I don't understand why I couldn't get any answers. Soon, I was too much of a wreck to think clearly enough about what to do.

I called my husband at work in tears. I told him what had happened and that since it was Friday I was afraid that I wouldn't be able to get anything done about Dan's eyes before the weekend - again. I asked him to call the eye center since sometimes a male voice got more things done.

Luckily my husband was able to go through the family doctor to get some information. They were told to just go to the ophthalmology clinic tomorrow and "Someone should be able to take a look at him"

So Saturday morning, I sent Dan and my husband to the eye clinic. I know that I am usually in charge of the specialists, but I was too emotional to make this trip.

When the afternoon rolled around and they hadn't returned I called my husband. Sam said, "We are next in line, but kids keep coming in with more serious eye emergencies."

They finally returned home late in the evening. Dan was super done with doctors after that.

"The doctor said that he has uveitis and that we were lucky it was the painful variety. Silent inflammation does the most damage because you don't know anything is wrong."

The doctor gave Dan steroid eye drops to calm the inflammation. He also said it was important to keep Dan's eyes dilated to protect his vision from permanent damage from the inflammation.

18 NEW EYE DOCTOR

The on-call ophthalmologist made sure Dan got an appointment with the pediatric ophthalmologist within the week. This doctor confirmed the diagnosis.

"Thirty years ago, Dan would probably have ended up a blind, cripple."

"New medicine is great," I agree. It does not come free though. I had no idea what this new development would cost.

The eye doctor made notes in Dan's chart.

"Do we really have to keep Dan's eyes dilated all the time?" I asked. The dilated eyes made Dan uncomfortable. I sympathized because I am useless for nearly the entire day if I have my eyes dilated for an eye exam.

"Yes it protects his vision while the eyes are swollen."

"How long will he have to do that?"

"It could be months."

I sighed. I had hoped eye-dilation was temporary because it seemed like a cruel thing to do to someone. Dan couldn't read and he wouldn't go outside because the bright light hurt his eyes.

"I'm going to refer you to a uveitis specialist. You are lucky because he is the premiere authority on uveitis. He writes textbooks on it."

I nodded. I was excited to have a famous doctor as long as he wasn't too busy to get an appointment with. Maybe he could figure out how to help Dan. I was tired of the wait-and-see approach.

Dan's first appointment at Dr. V's office was intimidating. The office was crowded and he needed lots of tests. It took 3 hours before we even saw the doctor.

Dr. V was soft-spoken and somewhat awkward, but I could tell he knew what he was doing. He became my favorite doctor.

"Enbrel can sometimes cause uveitis as a side-effect," he said. "Especially if you have been on Enbrel and then stopped."

"He was on Enbrel a few years ago and it really helped a lot. It is not helping him now though. Is there anything else available?"

"You can switch to something else. I think you should use Humira."

"Is that an injection?"

"Yes, but you only need to use it every 2 weeks."

"What about methotrexate?"

"Keep taking the methotrexate. The biologics work better when you use them with methotrexate."

I listened as carefully as I could. I hoped Dr. V would tell this to the rheumatologist because I had been getting the impression that Enbrel was the only choice.

"Until the swelling in his eyes go down, you should use stronger eye drops. They are more expensive, but you don't have to use them as often."

I took the prescriptions for eye drops that he gave me.

"Hopefully you will feel better soon, OK?" he said as he shook Dan's hand and then mine.

I love that he talked to Dan like his pain mattered.

19 HUMIRA

After the diagnosis of uveitis, I made an appointment with the rheumatologist. His name was Dr. Z and he seemed almost excited that Dan had a rare eye complication.

He looked at Dan's chart that had now been computerized.

"So Dan has developed uveitis."

"Yes, and his joints are still painful."

Dr. Z examined Dan's painful joints. Then he looked at Dan's eyes with a small light. The light made Dan flinch and blink.

"Is he taking eye drops?"

"Yes, prednisone drops and some drops to dilate his eyes."

Dr. Z made more notes as he said, "Dr. V says we need to change to Humira."

I was so excited that the doctor was considering different treatment. I wondered if we would have changed anything without the uveitis complication.

"Humira injections can sting," he explained.

"More than Enbrel?" I was thinking of how long Dan took to finish an injection of Enbrel.

"Yes," the doctor said.

I looked at Dan to see if he was listening. He was focusing on putting his shoes on. I hoped he hadn't heard the information about Humira.

"If you apply a lidocaine patch a few hours before the shot, it might help. Do you want to try that?"

"Yes, please," I said. Really, was there any other answer to that question?

Dr. Z was about to leave the exam room. But I was able to ask about payment assistance before he left. I did not leave the clinic without that information.

The payment assistance was based on a reimbursement. I was given card that was like a credit card, but it only had money after the receipts were submitted.

As with all health care, I knew that you wouldn't know how much something would cost until you actually ordered it. Then the drug companies negotiated with the insurance and then they played some kind of dart game that came up with a price we would be quoted at the medical pharmacy.

I held myself together as the pharmacist asked for $1200 for the month supply. I was so glad that all the cost would eventually be reimbursed because that was the same amount as our mortgage payment at the time.

I couldn't help thinking about the $600 vial of medicine that I handed to an 11-year-old. I hovered over him as he gave himself the injection because I was afraid he might drop the liquid gold. I guess I thought I would be able to make some kind of diving catch before it would shatter on the kitchen floor.

I helped Dan apply the lidocaine patch before the bi-weekly injections, but the shots were still painful.

Dan insisted on slowness, even slower than the Enbrel.

Injections could last hours.

20 FINDING METHOTREXATE

It was quite difficult to keep track of all Dan's medications especially since I had to go to different pharmacies to get them. I asked the doctor about cutting out methotrexate.

Dr. V, the ophthalmologist, said I needed to keep giving Dan methotrexate because it helps the Humira work better. If Dan takes both the methotrexate and Humira, then Dan would be less likely to build up a tolerance to the medication.

Armed with this information, I was determined to get all the medication Dan needed. I usually got the methotrexate at the same place as I obtained the Humira. But a few times the pharmacy told me they didn't have any.

"It's a countrywide shortage," the pharmacist told me when I looked at her like that was crazy. How can a pharmacy be out of a medicine like methotrexate?

After looking all over my local area, it turned out to be true. I couldn't find it (anywhere that my insurance covered it anyway)

I called different hospitals to try to locate it. One pharmacist told me they expected to get the next shipment within 4 weeks. At one point I had called all the pharmacies on our insurance plan. No one had the drug. This is when my panic mode kicked in.

I thought that maybe the rheumatology clinic had a secret stash. As usual, I had a hard time getting answers from them. Maybe because they deal with whiny patients all the time, they are not good at returning calls. The voice mail phone tree does not even have an option to ask a question. When the nurse finally called me back, she said "I've heard it can be hard to find, but just keep calling around."

So I kept calling around. I found a hospital that had one vial left so I dropped everything to go and get it. I suspect that they finally got off their butts and actually looked through their stock when they realized they had a frantic woman on the other end of the phone.

Eventually I had to give up on insurance-approved pharmacies. Walgreens usually had it and it was sometimes under $20. The prices always fluctuated for unknown reasons. After this problem with the shortage, I stockpiled the stuff just in case. I probably still have some in the house somewhere.

21 FUNDING

I'm going to take a break from our story to rant about how expensive a child with a chronic disease can be.

We started this journey around 2007. Our family had good insurance the entire time. We've had insurance since before Dan was diagnosed. Each year the deductible, co-pays and out-of-pocket maximum increased until we were paying $12,000/year in addition to our medical premiums that were also around $12,000/year. That is until the ACA. Thanks, Obama.

My husband makes a decent living, but in our 4th year of treatment, our budget was a mess. Our credit cards were maxed. Our house and cars were in disrepair. We ate from church welfare and got our clothes at the thrift store. Our furniture and toys were all from charity. We eventually had to go through bankruptcy. Medical bills are the largest cause of bankruptcy so I know we are not alone.

I wanted to help Dan, but I also resented the fact that his treatments kept us in virtual poverty.

"Can we go to the movies?" the kids asked me.

"I'm sorry we don't have any funding," I told them. I called it funding instead of money because I hoped to insulate them from the problems. Funding sounds like we are some kind of business just waiting for the expenses to be approved.

Not one of my family members stepped in to help, even though they could have. I felt abandoned which has really damaged our relationship and I don't think it will ever recover.

Life was so hard.

I worked part-time and took care of five high-maintenance children. Each of Dan's sisters also has their own special issues from clinical depression to chronic headaches. I worried that I couldn't give them the things they needed.

I was riddled with anxiety and self-doubt. I remember one night, I locked my bedroom door, curled up on my floor and just cried. I felt like my family and neighbors were judging me. I felt like God had abandoned me. I was a good person so why couldn't I catch a break. Why couldn't my family catch a break? All I saw ahead of me was on stressful situation after another. It would have been nice to end it all, but my kids needed me. I would not let them down.

Here is one example of how I felt so drained.

We got church assistance for food, but only after going through a difficult approval process every 2 weeks. I would fill out a form for things we needed and it had to be approved by two different church leaders. There were no easy-prep things on the list. I had to spend so much time cooking in order to make the food work for us. I felt like I couldn't even control what our family ate. And every time I asked for help, the leaders took the opportunity to judge me.

"You should focus more on Dan," one leader told me.

"I have to think of my other kids too," I explained.

"Maybe you could take Dan swimming more often, that will help with his joints," one advised me like they knew something about Dan's illness.

"I don't have time,"

"You need to make the time," they scolded.

"Of course," I said, agreeing just to get the interview over with.

I was doing the best I could but it was never good enough. If I had been good enough, my children would be cured, we would have money and we all would be happier.

22 MRI

Dan was on Humira for almost a year. His uveitis had subsided, but his ankles were still painful. He couldn't run or walk much. He always used crutches to walk short distances. He heavily leaned on me as I helped him up and down the stairs in our 60's era, multi-level house. I lugged around an old, heavy wheelchair when I took him out.

But now we had to switch to a different provider at the rheumatology clinic, a NP-C.

At this appointment, I had wheeled Dan into the exam room using the old, borrowed wheelchair. I told her that Dan's ankles were especially painful this past month.

She examined Dan's ankles.

"I don't see any swelling. He shouldn't be in pain." She said.

"But he can't walk for more than a few feet. He always uses crutches or a wheelchair."

"He shouldn't be using a wheelchair. Maybe you should be tougher on him."

Did she think I was lugging this 50 pound wheelchair around for fun?

I always tried to defer to the doctors at appointments. What did I really know? But this time I felt like I was being attacked because I was trying to help Dan get around easier.

There were days when I felt like the meanest mom in the world because I made him walk anywhere.

"I should make him walk even if it makes his pain worse?" I clarified.

I never felt like this nurse listened to me or Dan.

She looked over Dan's chart.

"I guess we could try an MRI," she finally offered like she was trying to placate a whiny child.

I scheduled the MRI as soon since it was near the end of the "insurance" year and we had already hit the high deductible on our plan.

I was excited that the MRI might prove to the nurse that Dan was actually in pain. Then maybe we could get a different treatment than Humira.

On the day of the MRI, I brought Dan to the children's hospital in his wheelchair. He got an IV so for contrast dye. He was such a pro at needle sticks; he didn't even make a fuss.

I sat outside the MRI room and listened to the machine pound away for nearly an hour while it analyzed Dan's ankles. Dan wore multi-media glasses and earphones so he didn't even hear the noises from the machine.

23 REMICADE

Dan and I went back to the clinic a few weeks after the MRI study. I was anxious to hear what the doctor would learn about his ankles.

"The MRI does show a tiny bit of swelling in the ankles," she said as if unimpressed.

"OK," I calmly said. Told ya!, I said in my head.

"I think we could switch Dan to Remicade."

"Is that another type of injection?"

"It is a medicine given as an IV infusion only. You have to go to the hospital for a few hours while they give the medicine."

I was ready to do anything to help Dan, so I quickly agreed to change his medication. It was the end of the year and we had already reached the out-of-pocket maximum.

"You get to go watch movies for a few hours," she told Dan.

"Is there a payment assistance program?" I asked. She gave me a folder of information on the program.

I left that appointment with more hope than I had felt in a long time. Maybe this change would work.

I called the hospital to arrange the new treatment.

"Can I schedule the infusion at a closer hospital" I asked the receptionist.

"Sure, we can do the infusion at that hospital on the children's floor."

She transfered me to another line and I made the appointment. I'm so glad we can go the hospital that is only 35 minutes away instead of 60 minutes. The shorter travel time and easier parking will make the appointment seem much shorter. So far it seems like things are working out well.

I filled out all the forms for payment assistance and faxed them where they were needed. I felt really prepared for this new experience.

24 FIRST REMICADE DOSE

When the day came for Dan's first dose of Remicade, we arrived at the usual rheumatology clinic. This confused the front desk. After many conversations, they realized we needed to go to the opposite side of the hospital - the South Tower. But the two places didn't connect.

"Go back to the first floor," the receptionist said as he pointed to the elevator. "Then follow the signs to the main hospital."

I pushed Dan's wheelchair as directed.

I wandered around the main hospital for a while. I soon became flustered when I couldn't find any sign of a children's floor. I started asking random people for help.

"Do you know where the children's floor is?" I asked a person at a pharmacy counter.

"No."

I found a gift shop and asked the clerk.

"Do you know where the children's floor is?"

"Try upstairs."

I finally found my way to the top floor of the South Tower. At the end of the hall, a double door is marked "Children's Floor" but was closed and locked.

I was almost ready to give up. I peaked through a small window in the door. It looked like a normal hospital floor.

There had to be people in there. Even if I was half an hour late, they had to let us in.

Then I noted and old-school phone on the wall.

I picked up the handset and heard ringing.

"I'm here for a Remicade infusion for my son," I said into the phone.

I heard papers shuffling and muffled voices before the doors jerked open.

The hospital floor was deserted except for a medical assistant that directed us to a room.

The assistant took Dan's vital signs and then I helped him from his wheelchair into a hospital bed.

I signed papers while they tried to talk to Dan.

"How are you feeling?"

"Fine."

Dan didn't answer. I'm sure the staff tries to make the kids feel more comfortable by talking to them. But Dan is not good at small talk.

On the other hand, I'm a pro at talking about nothing with medical assistants. The key is to give enough information to avoid awkward silence, but not enough information to cause alarm. Talking about the weather is always safe. I always try to appear normal and share just enough to help with medical care.

"What do you like to do?" the MA asked.

"He likes to play video games," I offered. This is not exactly the truth since we were too poor to own a game system. But it was a good non-offensive answer.

The MA gave Dan a binder open to a page listing many video games.

Dan put the list on the table without looking at it.

I could tell he is nervous, so I helped him choose a game, hoping it would distract him.

A few minutes later, the nurse bought medication in a small cup. She also gave him a juice box.

"Your orders say to start with Benadryl."

Dan swallowed the pill.

Then the nurse prepared Dan for the IV. They got all the supplies and raised up the bed so his hand was easier to reach.

Eleven-year-old Dan sat still while they tried three times to start the IV line. I think the nurse felt worse about it than Dan did. One nurse gave Dan a warm pack to put on his hand.

"If we get the blood flowing better, it might help," she said.

She called another nurse to help and they finally got the IV started.

When the nurses left the room to get the medicine, I asked Dan if it hurt.

"No," he said. He had finally started to play the video game.

About half an hour after the infusion started, Dan became too tired to play so we watched movies. He ate some lunch and watched more movies.

The first time they infused Remicade, they did it slowly to make sure there wasn't a reaction. After over 6 hours, Dan's only reaction was sleepiness and that was probably due to the Benadryl.

I was emotionally exhausted. I was not excited to do this again in only 2 weeks.

25 NEW DOCTOR

We went back to get another dose of Remicade at 2 weeks, 4 weeks and 6 weeks later.

After Dan finished that course of medication, we went back to the doctor to check in.

When we got to the clinic, we found we had been assigned to a new doctor again. This was our 5th rheumatologist.

I wheeled Dan into the exam room.

"How are you feeling?" Dr. B asked.

"Fine," Dan said. He has never admitted to much pain at the doctor's office. I think he gets nervous around the doctors especially as he had gotten older.

"He still has a lot of pain," I said. Why were we here if Dan feels fine?

"It can take a while for the Remicade to work."

This is the usual answer that I was expecting. And that is fine. But can we make our lives more comfortable in the meantime?

"Can we get a prescription or something for a better wheelchair?"

I don't think Dr. B hears me as he looks over Dan's chart. He always kind of squints as he tries to look through the bottom of his bifocal glasses.

When I don't get a response about the wheelchair, I figured I could find one on my own. Then I ask about a handicap parking pass.

Dr. B looks up. "I can get you papers for one of those. But continue to get the Remicade every 6 weeks."

"OK, thank you, " said as I take the papers that he gives to me.

While waiting for the medicine to start working, I jump through the hoops for the parking pass which means a trip to the county DMV to wait in line where I am grilled about my reasons for the pass. There must be people who park in handicap places without needing them. Trust me, I am not one of them.

I also find an online store that sells wheelchairs. I find the lightest one I can. It is so cheap because it is really like a big stroller since the wheelchair rider can't control it at all. I didn't figure I needed that feature since Dan's hands hurt too much to try making the chair move.

And then, much to my amazement, Dan started to improve and he didn't use the wheelchair as often. His uveitis was totally quiet and we stopped all eye drops.

We made our regular trips to the children's floor for infusions. All the nurses on the floor recognized Dan because we were there so often. The infusions continued to make Dan tired due to the Benadryl. I also still became exhausted due to the mental stress. I think hospitals just have that effect on me.

Once at the end of one infusion, Dan got a fever which made the nurse nervous. He was given some Tylenol and required to stay longer for observation. The Tylenol helped, but because of that reaction, the rest of the infusions had to be even slower than they had been taking.

Dan and I watched a lot of movies at the hospital. His favorite movies involved pirates or Harry Potter, all of which almost immediately put me to sleep.

26 INSURANCE WOES

I enrolled Dan in Remistart, a program to help pay for Remicade. The paperwork was annoying, but doable. And Dan was easily approved.

Unfortunately, the cost of the hospital administering the infusion was not covered. Each treatment cost us about $1200 after insurance and reimbursement. We met our high out-of-pocket maximum quickly.

I talked to the doctor about options.

"Could I get a nurse to come to our house to give the infusion there?" I asked. "The hospital bills are so high."

"I wish you could, but the medication is too risky. Dan has already had a reaction."

Dan's eye doctor, the fabulous and famous specialist in uveitis was not in our approved insurance network. Every visit hit us with a $150 which we didn't have.

I tried to explain the issue to my insurance company which was a scary thing to do because it is so hard to even figure out who to talk to.

"Dr. V is the only doctor who treats uveitis in my state. Other doctors won't even look at Dan. They will send us to Dr. V"

"OK ma'am. I will have to call 3 random ophthalmologists and ask if they treat uveitis."

"I've already done that, trust me. He is the only one in the state."

"I'm sorry, ma'am. It is policy."

"I've really had it with this," I said as my voice starts to crack with emotion. I hate how I can get so emotional when I talk to stupid insurance companies. This person I'm talking to on the phone is just a cog in the giant machine that is the healthcare system.

"Awww, honey, don't worry. I'll call you back real soon."

The fact that she said that so me was so surprising. I had been lucky enough to find a person that sounded like she cared.

"OK, thank you," I said quietly.

After hanging up, I had to walk around the block a few times to cool off.

The insurance representative called me back within the hour.

"Dr. V has been approved for 90 days. Then you will have to get another exception."

"That's great news. Thank You."

It wasn't great news, because it meant I would have to go through this for every visit to Dr. V since Dan had to follow up every 90 days. I tried to get all the paperwork done as best I could, but it never seemed to work out. The eye clinic still charged us the same amount so I gave up on the in-network status for Dr. V.

27 SCOUTS

Dan is now about 12-years-old. This is the time that all the neighbors at church were expected to participate in boy scouts. I wanted Dan to be part of the boys, but I didn't let him participate in camp-outs. If he slept outside on the cold ground, his pain would be worse for days.

I once sent him to a camp-out to see if it would work out. I make him take a padded cot to sleep on. I had bought it especially to see if we could make camping work. When the scout leaders saw the cot they said that he didn't need to take so many things. After a few more comments about my inability to parent, I reluctantly let him attend the camp-out. But that was the last time.

The bishop of the ward called me to discuss the situation. They did not like that Dan skipped camping. If he didn't go on enough camp-outs, he would never achieve the rank of Eagle; as if getting an Eagle scout award is the only thing that matters.

"You need to cut those apron strings. Boys need these experiences."

"He is too sick."

"He doesn't seem sick to me. I've seen him run and play with the other boys."

I wasn't surprised to hear that. Dan likes to be with his friends and sometimes will push himself more than he should because he is only 12. He may look like a man, but he is still a child.

"But you don't see what happens after that. He limps around the house for days until he recovers."

"He is just playing you."

Even if he was, it was still my call. I seethed in my head, but didn't say it out loud. I wish I had said something out loud.

"No he isn't," I said. I didn't know what else to say if the bishop wasn't going to believe me anyway. Maybe I could help him understand.

"He takes high-power medicine to help treat his auto-immune disease. His medicine makes him immunosuppressed which means he is more susceptible to infections." We didn't really have that much trouble with infections, but more than a few times we have gotten antibiotics for scrapes that started to look scary. So I may have exaggerated a little, but I don't think the guy was following me anyway - too many medical terms.

"I didn't know that," he said.

And I think, of course you didn't know that. No one ever cares to ask about his disease. They judge first and then ask questions later.

"I know you want the best for him, but I've been dealing with this for years. It makes no sense, but overexertion makes the pain worse the next day."

"If you have enough faith, it will all work out."

My faith was failing and it wasn't working out.

The best thing that had worked out for Dan was for me to stand up for him.

28 IMPROVEMENT

I really don't know what caused Dan's improvement this time. Was it the medicine, the exercise or just good luck for a change?

I cheered when we put the wheelchair and crutches in the shed after they went unused for months.

I was able to make him do more homework without feeling guilty since he could use his hands fully. His handwriting improved.

I even signed him up for violin lessons. His stiff fingers had a hard time at first, but he improved so much. He sometimes complained that his ankles hurt to stand and play so I convinced his teachers to let him sit during lessons.

"Why are you watching me practice the violin," Dan asked while he practiced one evening.

"Remember when you couldn't even move your fingers because of arthritis? That's why I love to watch you play."

Dan rolled his eyes at me for that.

When he turned twelve, he had a growth spurt. He was 6 feet tall with a deep voice. All the hospital nurses thought he was at least 16-years-old. He love to hear them say that.

The summer after he turned twelve, he felt well enough to go to week-long scout camp.

I agreed to let him go since he had been walking better and his Dad was going to go with him for some of the days.

I was proud to attend the award ceremony after camp and saw his friends get 4 or 5 merit badges.

"Why did you only get 2 merit badges?" I asked Dan.

"My ankles hurt too much to get to the classes," he said.

I guess he wasn't as better as I thought he was.

29 MORE IMPROVEMENT

After I realized that Dan was not pain-free. I thought maybe a little exercise loosen up his joints. If I could get him moving he might feel better. He used to do karate and soccer, but had to drop out of those due to pain.

"What do you like to do?"

"Ice skating," he said.

I think he said that because he knew I wouldn't keep up with that. The closest rink was a 30 minute drive away. We could go once in awhile, but not enough to get meaningful exercise.

"What is your second choice?"

"Swimming."

Did he know I didn't like swimming? The pool was only 10 minutes away and would be much more doable. I called his bluff and bought a family pass to the local pool and made swimming practice a priority.

We made it to the rec center two or three times a week. Dan and I swam a few laps while his younger sisters played in the shallow end. I don't know if the swimming made a difference, but it made me feel like I was doing something to help Dan's joints.

As I get older I think that regular exercise has kept me sane and healthy and I was hoping to instill the love of exercise in

Dan. I don't know if that worked, but by the next summer he was able to fully participate in the week-long scout camp and had the time of his life moving and playing like a normal boy.

30 ANOTHER FLARE-UP

Dan was symptom free for almost a year. He rode his bike, walked and played outside without problems. He even hiked through Disneyland for 5 days that summer.

The rheumatologist tapered Dan off all arthritis medication. I was hopeful but nervous since we had done this before.

Two months later, Dan says, "Mom, I have bad news. My knee is swollen again."

I called the doctor who put Dan back on methotrexate and anti-inflammatories. But the medicine didn't stop Dan's knees, wrists and other joints from continuing to swell.

At one point he had a hard time bending his knees enough to get into the car.

Dr. B saw Dan when his joints were the worst they had been in years. He gave him a high dose of prednisone and increased the methotrexate 50%. He also prescribed a medicine to help with mouth sores: leucovorin. The leucovorin was much more effective at preventing mouth sores than the folic acid ever was. I wish we could have had that medicine years ago.

The prednisone helps ease Dan's pain and swelling, but not enough. Dr. B prescribed Remicade infusions again.

It surprised me that it took three months for my insurance company to agree to cover the medication. This was exactly the same medicine he used to be on when we had the same insurance.

At one office visit, I asked Dr. B why it took so long.

"I don't know," he answered, "insurance said it was not a usual treatment for arthritis. I sent a letter explaining Dan's history and eight journal articles for them to read." I loved Dr. B.

Due to Dr. B's influence, we finally got insurance approval. Dan received Remicade infusions every four weeks. We got them at the children's hospital again. I felt kind of silly bringing my giant 15-year-old son to the children's hospital. Eventually the insurance had a fit about the pricey hospital infusions and demanded we take Dan to an infusion center.

I found and infusion center which would accept the orders and the insurance. I was excited about this change because I hate hospitals. The infusion center would also be much closer, quicker and less expensive than the hospital.

The nurses at the infusion center were so nice and made us feel special and lucky to be there. They were really good at getting Dan's IV started. In the past he would have to suffer through 3 or 4 attempts to get a line started. The infusion nurses always got the vein on the first try. They also gave him as much Dr. Pepper as he could drink.

The Remicade, methotrexate and other anti-inflammatories helped get the flare-up under control and Dan was able to start 11th grade the next fall with no problems. He even earned straight A's on his college level classes.

Sometimes when the weather changes, his joint pain will flare up, but the rheumatologist will prescribe a short course of prednisone which can help Dan feel better.

The summer after 11th grade, Dan was doing so well that Dr. B thought we could taper a little bit on the medicine, but to keep most things the same. I agree that I don't want to stop the current treatment because it makes it harder to keep the pain flares under control.

31 MORE UPS AND DOWNS

Dan is now leaving for college. He graduated level 10 of Suzuki violin. He earned his associates degree while in High School and got a great scholarship to a state university. He has a job working with children at a space simulation camp. He can probably go anywhere or do anything he wants. This future is quite different than the one that use to haunt me as a young mother. I feared that he would regret all the things he missed. I imagined him living in my basement, depressed, playing video games and blaming me for his problems.

Being a child with juvenile arthritis is the only thing that Dan knows. If it changed him in anyway it was to make him stronger. He has a great attitude. He is smart and compassionate especially for people who deal with chronic disease. He is my one child who always remembers to take his medicine without any reminders.

My favorite nurse told me that the reason that Dan was able to do so many things --from playing the violin, to having a job and doing so well at school was because he had a mother who worked so hard to take care of him. And maybe for the first time I believed it because she had seen a lot of patients with his condition and always remarked that he was doing so well. I teared up because being the mother of a child with a chronic disease it one of the hardest, thankless jobs around.

32 LESSONS

I learned a lot as I took care of my son with juvenile arthritis. I learned to call doctors and insurance companies. I learned how to buy expensive medicine and cheap wheelchairs. I learned that you have to be the voice for your child.

5 things I learned from parenting a child with arthritis.
1. It's not your fault. Bad things happen for no reason.
2. Enjoy every good day
3. Stand up for your child
4. Expensive medication are miracles
5. Alternative medicine is nice, but many times not the answer.

5 things that made the most difference to Dan's quality of life:
1. Keep life as normal as possible
2. Chiropractic care. Kind of alternative medicine, but it was just to make him more comfortable, not a cure.
3. Crutches or wheelchairs when needed.
4. Believe when they say they are in pain.
5. Don't be afraid to ask questions. When Dan developed chronic headaches I didn't think there were any other pain drugs he could take. He was already on a high dose of NSAID's.

The doctor prescribed Amitriptyline, an antidepressant that can prevent headaches. It helped Dan's quality of life so much.

Here are top 5 things that I wish I had done.
1. Stopped blaming myself.
2. Stopped wishing that he could be like other kids
3. I wish I had bought a house without stairs.
4. I wish I had been better as asking the right questions.
5. I wish I had insisted on professional therapy for me.

33 MEDICATIONS

Nonsteroidal anti-inflammatory drugs (NSAID)

These drugs work against the chemicals that cause inflammation. Dan used Anaprox (naproxen sodium) Feldene (piroxicam) and Mobic (meloxicam) at different times. I liked Mobic because you only need to take it once a day. If these drugs are taken long-term, you need to watch for the side effects with blood tests.

Glucocorticoids:

If the NSAIDs don't help, a rheumatologist may try a round of prednisone. This can help with flare-ups. But not good for long term use.

Disease-modifying anti-rheumatic drugs (DMARDs)

Methotrexate: This drug is used to treat cancer because it interferes with cell reproduction, especially fast-reproducing cells like cancer cells or bone marrow cells. Since it lowers the amount of blood cells it also lowers the amount of immune cells. This can reduce the amount of cells that might attack your own body including your joints. So this is why it is helpful for rheumatoid arthritis and other autoimmune arthritis conditions. This drug was first invented in the 1940's so it is a pretty cheap drug. It is given as a shot or as pills once a week.

Vitamins

If you are taking methotrexate, you should be taking folic acid. Since methotrexate affects the folic acid synthesis pathway, patients who take this drug may become deficient which can produce some nasty side-effects including nausea and mouth sores. I'm not convinced this helped much with Dan's side-effects, it always made the doctors feel better if he was taking it. Leucovorin is a stronger version of folic acid that work on a different step of the folic acid synthesis pathway. It works really well at preventing the mouth-sores (like canker sores) that are super painful.

Biologic Response Modifiers:

These are the expensive ones, but the drugs that seem to have the most effectiveness at stopping the disease. They are usually given as shots or IV infusions. The shots are not pleasant because they can sting when they are administered. Some varieties of these are Enbrel (etanercept), Humira (adalimumab) and Remicade (infliximab). I later learned that it is best to be on methotrexate while on one of these drugs to prevent resistance.

Headache medicine:

Dan developed horrible headaches when he was about 12 and since he was already taking so many pain drugs for his arthritis, I didn't know what to give him. Luckily amitriptyline helped to prevent the worst headaches.

SUPPORT

Thank you for listening to my story. If you have any questions our would like to chat, send me an email at dianekir@gmail.com